CAREGIVING BASICS: HELP FOR NEW CAREGIVERS

By

Robert Grice, Ph.D., LPC

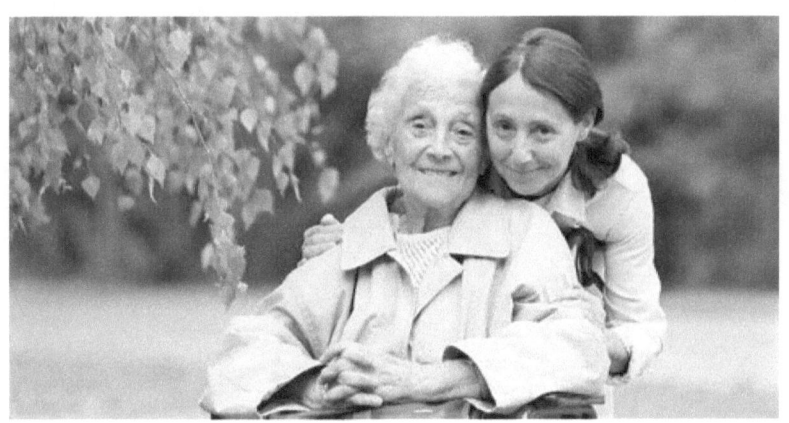

Contents

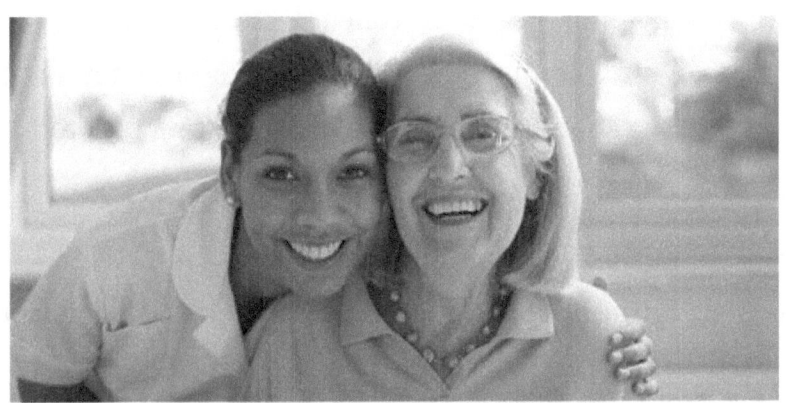

Introduction

The need to provide caregiving for a family member eventually touches most families. Volunteering to be a caregiver for others is a noble task, but it can become an exhausting task too.

The *negative* implications include health problems, relationship problems, and health issues. Burnout does not occur overnight. The condition begins with ignoring warning signs of trouble.

Research has revealed several actions that tend to improve the quality of caregiving and the overall quality of life of the caregiver. We know methods are available to enhance caregiving.

1. Remember, you can do this!

2. Be as informed as possible.

3. Practice self-care

4. Monitor Your Self-Talk

5. Engage in Planning and Goal setting

6. Learn to Communicate

7. Managing Stress

Is Family Caregiving an Issue?

Statistics from 2015 and published by the Family Caregiver Alliance indicate that 43.5 million Americans have provided unpaid caregiving services. Most are not healthcare professionals and are called *informal caregivers*.[1] The value of those services was $470 million in 2013.

Volunteering for Service

Martha called her mother repeatedly one morning, only to reach her answering machine. Martha's mother generally answered with the second ring. Martha's mother always answered the phone if she was home.

Martha knew she was not away from home. Worried that something might be wrong, Martha traveled across town to her mother's house and found her on the kitchen floor. Her mother had a stroke at some point and could not move.

Martha's world changed that day. Martha's mother survived but was bedridden following the

---

[1] https://www.caregiver.org/resource/caregiver-statistics-demographics/

incident. Martha was an only child, and she had no one else to call upon to help take care of her mother. Martha's plans of taking a vacation the following month suddenly faded away. Her daughter had a school play that weekend, but now Martha would not attend.

Martha's husband planned a special romantic dinner at a local restaurant where reservations had to be made weeks in advance. He would need to reschedule those reservations. Martha would likely either move in with her mother or move her mother in with her family.

Martha's story may sound extreme, but it frequently happens when family members or close friends unexpectedly take on the role of caregiver. The task is complex, and they are often unprepared. Most caregivers lack medical training, which requires a learning curve, plus they must learn the patient's schedule.

The caregiver will become familiar with stress. Unexpected setbacks can be traumatic. They often experience dwindling support and contact with others with time, and people tend to forget the homebound and those who care for them. Stress on the caregiver's family grows as the caregiver is forced to withdraw from many social interactions.

Sadly, the health of caregivers often suffers. Their relationships may begin to break down. Physical problems tend to increase with persistent stress and not care for themselves. Psychological distress is expected in response to the pressure of being responsible for someone else and experiencing trauma with unexpected setbacks like the patient's admittance to the hospital.

Can we offer suggestions to help new caregivers minimize the impact of caregiving on their lives and families?

Yes, the following are suggestions that can help caregivers remain healthy in every way while serving someone else.

#1 Remember, You Can Do This!

The first recommendation is to be confident. You can do this! Will it be easy? Probably not and learning new skills and information can be a challenge, but you can do it. You may feel overwhelmed at first, but the practice has a way of training us in new skills and knowledge.

I know the mere thought of all you must now know can be overwhelming. New medical knowledge could include:

- Learning to deal with feeding tubes
- Giving shots
- Providing breathing treatments
- Feed the patient
- Bathe the patient
- Assist with personal hygiene
- Make doctor appointments
- Provide transportation to medical appointments
- Accompany to medical appointments
- Confer with doctors
- Administer medication

- Pick up medication from the pharmacy
- Wound treatments
- Physical therapy

Practical assistance with other tasks includes:

- Managing the patient's finances and legal issues
- Deal with any crisis that arises
- Serve as host for visitors
- Caring for the house
- Buying groceries and cooking
- Provide companionship
- Serve as a full-time aide
- Provide laundry services

What if you feel confused? If you have questions, ask someone. Numerous resources are available to help with caregiving. For instance, The Family Caregiver Alliance (FCA) offers various resources that cover every aspect of caregiving and identifies additional resources that could prove helpful.[2]

---

[2] https://www.caregiver.org/caregiving-101-being-caregiver

What if you feel overwhelmed? That's okay. Most people do at some point. We usually think overwhelmed when too much comes at us simultaneously, and much of it feels out of our control.

What can new caregivers do to overcome feeling overwhelmed? The **Family Caregiver Alliance** offers the following recommendations:

- Identify as a caregiver or embrace the role.
- Get a proper diagnosis even if from more than one doctor
- Learn the skills associated with their diagnosis
- Clarify the patient's finances, legal, and healthcare issues
- Have legal paperwork (e.g., wills, powers of attorney) in order
- Confer with the immediate family and others involved in the patient's life so that everyone remains on the same page.
- Identify and connect with resources and support in your community.

Planning can go a long way in mitigating the symptoms of stress that overwhelm us. Clarity, communication, and community are three powerful tools to help us maintain our sanity in the wake of stress and setbacks. So, remember that you are competent, and you can do this.

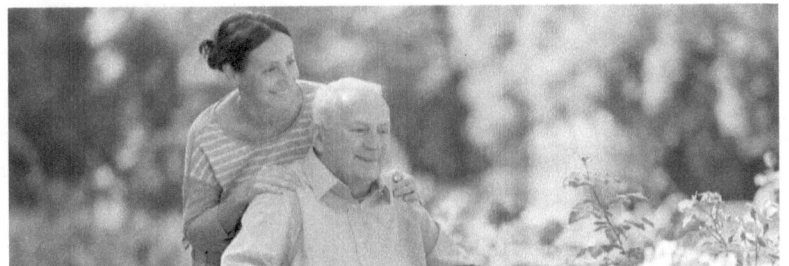

#2 Be as Informed As Possible.

"Knowledge is power" is a famous saying and a true statement. Knowing what to expect can be a powerful way to maintain your sanity when the caregiving situation becomes overwhelming. Sometimes caregivers may work with a client where recovery is likely and probable.

The information required might be more in-depth at the beginning when the situation is most involved. Still, as the caregiver becomes more familiar with providing care and with the patient's needs, the severity of the experience decreases, and less information may be required.

The opposite applies to those patients not likely to recover. Situations where the patient's condition will decline over time, require more information. For instance,

- What are the possible physiological changes?
- What cognitive changes will appear?
- Will the client become incontinent as the disease progresses?

- What equipment will likely be needed as the client's condition worsens?
- Will the client lose the ability to communicate?
- Will we need to see specialists in the future?
- Is hospitalization likely as part of this disease?
- Will the client feed, groom, or dress without assistance?
- What knowledge will be needed as the client's condition worsens?
- What new medication might we need?
- Will the patient's condition likely reach the point that home care is no longer possible?
- Should I expect behavioral changes?
- How much patient money is available for care? Is the balance sufficient? If not, where will they find the money?
- How long does the patient likely have left?

#3 Practice Self-Care

Self-care is imperative in every work that involves helping others. How good are you at taking care of yourself? How much time do you devote to making deposits in your revitalization each week? Caregivers must watch the warning signs of exhaustion or burnout, or they can inflict significant harm on the patient.

As a counselor, I often ask clients what they do in self-care. I often receive a blank stare in response accompanied by the remark, "What is that?"

The fact is we can quickly get too busy doing good and needful things, and we do so at the expense of our bodies, minds, and relationships.

A principle often overlooked is that what happens to the patient often happens to the caregiver. In other words, where the patient goes, the caregiver must go.

Suppose the patient is in the hospital and the caregiver is with the patient. In that case, the caregiver feels like a patient. They are often confined to the hospital room and may experience the same stress as the patient. The result is these caregivers face higher rates of depression and anxiety and decreases in quality of life.

Though most caregivers are female, the potential personal implications of caregiving tend to afflict males and females alike. The problems arise due to sleep deprivation, weak or absent self-care, and ignoring their illnesses, including putting off making medical appointments for themselves.

Caregivers are at risk of turning to substances like alcohol, tobacco, or other drugs as a method for dealing with stress. By some estimates, 46 to 59 percent report persistent depression.[3] While some caregivers may require medical intervention, most may find relief merely by engaging in self-care.

What is self-care? I use the analogy of a bank account with clients. Everyone has an internal bank account. Whenever we encounter some stressor, or others draw energy and effort, we write checks on that account.

---

[3] https://www.caregiver.org/taking-care-you-self-care-family-caregivers

At some point, if we make no deposits, we will be overdrawn. When someone becomes emotionally "overdrawn," nothing is left, and all the positivity we expect is gone. We begin to shut down with no fuel, much like an engine with an empty fuel tank.

What is self-care? In one sense, there are multiple answers to this question because what constitutes self-care for one may not be significant for another.

Self-Care is those attitudes and actions that enrich and reinvigorate our lives. They recharge our physical and psychological batteries. In doing so, they help us manage our relationships.

What are some common self-care attitudes and actions?

- The first step in self-care is recognizing that the caregiver is responsible for their self-care.
- Know your limitations
- Avoiding perfectionism because the goal is impossible
- Properly managing and expressing emotions – We deal with them, or they deal with us.

- Be honest about depression and anxiety – Ignoring the problem does not make the pain disappear.
- Have realistic expectations of yourself, the patient, and others.
- Avoid operating on assumptions and presumptions
- Identify and practice coping skills
- Establish healthy boundaries and learn to say "no."
- Avoid the martyr complex by keeping your service in perspective.
- Identify your stressors.
- Let's get physical – Find some exercise or activity that you enjoy (e.g., walking, running)
- Eat right – What you eat is the food you use.
- Get plenty of sleep – Tired caregivers become grumpy caregivers (7-8 hours)
- Accept help from others
- Try to find relief so you can take regular breaks
- Remain involved in your family.

The issue of self-care always raises questions about selfishness. Is it selfish to take care of ourselves when doing so might take away from our concern for others? Associating self-care with selfishness is a way to motivate guilt by accusing people of not doing enough in caregiving.

Self-care is not selfish; self-care is survival. I do not know your experience, but I have been around caregivers who ignored their need for self-care and gave until they gave out.

What happened next? They became cynical, critical, and apathetic. Why? They had nothing left to draw upon as fuel for caregiving.

The FCA offers multiple resources and suggestions of ways to practice self-care. For instance, the Caregiving Issues and Strategies page offers recommendations or tips for caregiver respite and techniques to make these breaks possible.[4]

The point is that the individual is still responsible for their self-care as a caregiver. The lack of self-care can put the caregiver in need of a caregiver. One resource that can be helpful is the Family Caregiver Alliance. The organization can be reached at (800) 445-8106 to learn about local

---

[4]www.caregiver.org

services or visit www.caregiver.org and click on
"Family Care Navigator."

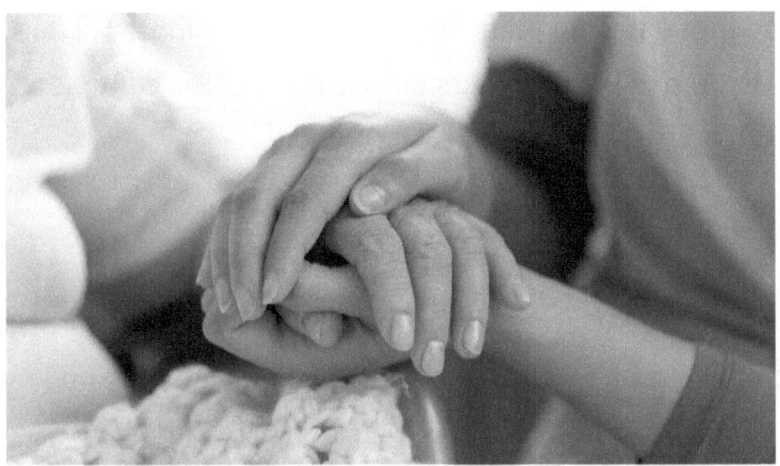

#4 Monitor Your Self-Talk

Self-talk is the inner conversation we rely upon to motivate and guide us in making decisions. The fact that our self-talk is ours does not mean the content of our self-talk is correct.

The content of self-talk can be false in reflecting reality, but we assume the content is accurate. Negative self-talk often reflects inaccurate information because it attacks personal ability and competency.

For instance, negative self-talk convinces us that whatever we attempt is doomed to failure. The failure is due to our incompetence or ineptness or due to the influence of others. All self-talk has a way of growing and expanding. Negative self-talk can lead to:

- Personalizing or self-blaming for everything
- Magnifying or only recognizing the negative characteristics or outcomes of our actions.
- Catastrophizing or assuming every situation will end in its worst possible scenario.

- Polarizing or resorting to black and white thinking assuming all is good or bad.

What are examples of negative self-talk?

- I can do it all by myself.
- If I do not care for the patient, no one will.
- If I do my best, others will love and appreciate me.
- Others will show appreciation for what I do.
- Keeping busy serving others will take my problems away.
- The family should always take care of its own.
- I always promised I would take care of my loved ones.
- My family will not mind if I am absent for a while.
- Caretaking should take priority over self-care.
- I must be perfect
- I must provide care to make up for what I did in the past.
- I will finally receive the patient's love and acceptance that I need.
- I am responsible for the patient's health.

- Stress is a normal part of life.
- I should make myself be a caregiver because that is what God would want me to do.
- A "real" Christian should want to provide care for the hurting.
- Self-care is selfish
- If I am not exhausted, I have not done my best caring for the patient.

The way to remedy stinking thinking is to practice self-honesty and embrace the truth. Caregiving is not easy, and we can make the experience worse if guided by inaccurate assumptions and ultimately imprison us in stress and despair.

What are the benefits of positive self-talk?[5] The overall benefit is positive self-talk produces optimism that we can be successful. Additionally, positive self-talk leads to...

- Greater satisfaction in life
- Improved cardiovascular health
- Increased sense of well-being
- Less stress

---

[5] https://www.healthline.com/health/positive-self-talk#benefits-of-self--talk

- Improved immune function
- Increased self-confidence
- Greater motivation to try

Caregiving is challenging, but positive self-talk is possible. Positive self-talk is essential to get through difficult times and setbacks. The key is that positive self-talk must be consistent. Therefore, positive self-talk is a habit and many times a habit we must develop in replacing negative self-talk.

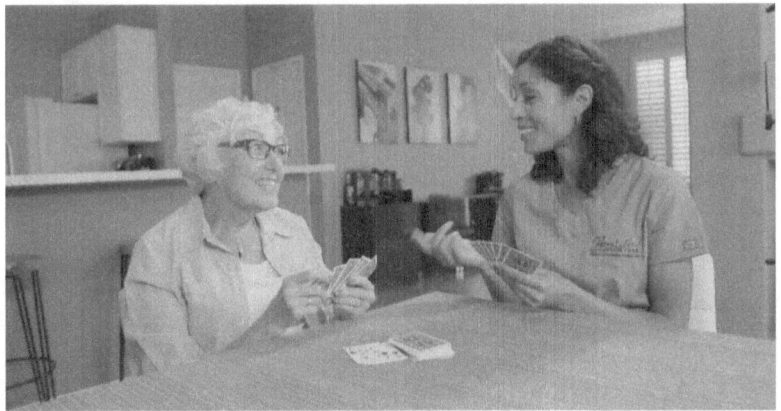

#5 Engage in Planning and Goal Setting

Once the caregiving process lasts longer than a few days, care pressures will surface along with weaknesses in the current care plan. These situations call for planning and goal setting.

Planning should focus on the quality of care foremost but must also consider efficiency and the current limitations such as resources and the training of caregivers.

Goal setting compliments the planning process by imposing specific parameters on the planning process. Anyone can plan anything, but having measurable goals puts those plans into action.

Setting goals requires more than wishful thinking or "should" and "oughts" to succeed. The best goals are measurable and accountable. In other words, what are your goals? Why are these goals important?

How will you hold yourself responsible for achieving these goals? How will you measure progress? Will you allow for partial fulfillment? Will you give yourself rewards for achieving the goals? What action steps are needed to achieve these goals?

Any number of goals are possible. Examples of goals include:

- Goals involving care.
- Setting aside time each week to take a break
- Securing help
- Holding regular communication sessions with the family
- Finding respite support
- Engaging in self-care activities
- Spending time each week with family

The SMART goals matrix is a simple and effective way to create goals with a high probability of achievement.

SMART Goals Criteria

S	Specific	What will be accomplished? Be precise and quantitative, if possible.
M	Measurable	How will progress be measured? What quantitative measurements are most appropriate?
A	Achievable	Can you achieve the goal? Is the goal achievable?
R	Relevant	Why is this goal important? How does the goal relate to the higher goals in your life?
T	Time-bound	What is the amount of time allowed to achieve this goal? Will there be checkpoints along the way?

Goal setting, at times, may be idealistic because conditions change. The good news is that goals can be revised if needed to reflect current circumstances.

However, deviating from a fundamental goal, such as engaging in self-care, should not be permanent. Resume pursuing the original goal as quickly as possible. If it was required, then it probably still is.

What is needed? Evaluate the situation. What were the current weaknesses in the care program or for the caregivers? What changes are required?

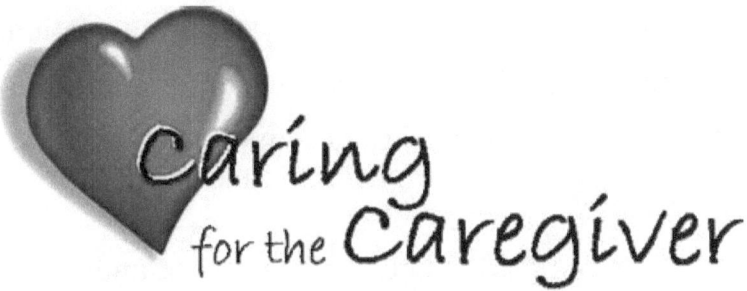

#6 Learn to Communicate

Communication is an essential part of the caregiving process. Everyone probably knows what assuming does to us when it comes to communication. The patient and caregiver must learn to communicate, and the caregiver must learn to communicate with the patient's family.

Communication between the patient and caregiver enables the two to be on the same therapeutic page. The patient and caregiver need to create their language. In time, they likely will be able to communicate verbally and nonverbally.

Both must understand the other. If the two do not communicate, the caregiver will not fully understand what the patient might be experiencing.

Communication between the caregiver and the family is critical in providing the optimum quality of care. Honesty is imperative, as well as communicating with the right attitude. Miscommunication is a constant threat as it leads to disputes and disagreements. When relationship problems arise, the primary attention must remain on clear communication that enhances the quality of care.

What are some ways to improve communication in the caregiving context? Focus on "I" statements when describing how you feel or what expectations were not met and avoid "you" statements. "You" statements always assign *blame* to others for one's own emotions. Blaming others might help us feel better, but the strategy seldom produces the positive outcomes that we seek.

Respect the feelings of others. Do not go out of your way to be rude or disrespectful. If your goal is to improve communication, this will not happen if the other person feels disrespected.

Try to see the other person's perspective. Sometimes others may be offensive due to something they perceive or something going on in their lives. For example, they may say something to the caregiver angrily, but their anger comes from something going on at home.

Be clear and specific in your communication. Do not make hints or implications and assume the other person will understand what you want to communicate. Be direct, be respectful, and be precise.

Lastly, be a good listener. Many times, we can avoid confusion and misunderstanding by merely saying nothing. Being a good listener is an invaluable trait.

Making Requests

Clear communication is necessary when asking for help. Caregivers can feel guilty about asking for help because they do not want to inconvenience or burden others or think others will not do a good job.

If you need help as the caregiver, ask for it. Have a specific list of ways in mind that others can help you. Be clear about what you want. Pay attention to the warning signs.

Is our patience wearing thin? The warning lights are flashing. Pay attention. Are you exhausted? If so, you are quickly moving towards burnout. It is entirely possible that a caregiver can cause more harm than good.

Ask for help. Consider the abilities of the ones you ask. Some may have the ability to cook and asking for help would be a natural fit. If you ask for help in an area of strength in the other person, they will be more likely to help.

Do not ask the same person for help every time. They may come to resent the caregiver and the request. True, relying on more than one or two people for support may be difficult due to the willingness of those at your disposal. The fact is that we tend to ask the same person or people every time for help because they said "yes" in the past.

Pick the best time to ask. Do not ask someone during stressful times or when distracted by other commitments. Wait until the person is relaxed and open to your request.

Be prepared for reluctance and refusal. Your request for help may not receive a warm reception. Our natural reaction is to become angry or to strike back at these "insensitive" people who do not care about the sacrifices we are making.

Others may respond with reluctance in that they respond with a generic "let me think about it" or "I will get back with you." If we press the issue, they may never help. If we leave it alone, the person might change their mind and help.

Avoid using ambiguity in your requests. A qualifier often sounds polite, but it weakens the request and gives the other person wiggle room to say "no."

When someone rejects our polite qualifier, the natural reaction is anger or to adopt a martyr mentality. Neither response is helpful. Be direct in your requests. If you need time off, do not make it negotiable.

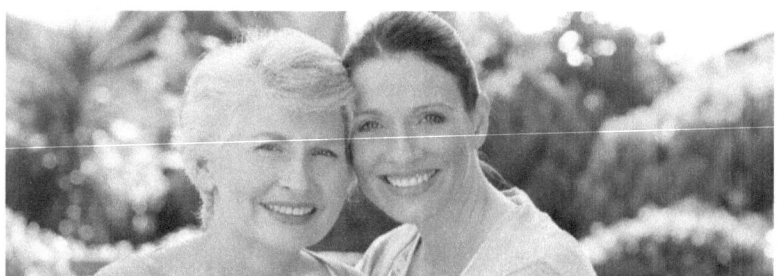

#7 Managing Stress

Effective caregiving over time requires we learn how to manage stress. What are the ways to manage stress?

- **Identify the sources of stress.** What are the stressors we face? What is causing my anxiety?
- **Monitor your emotions**. What is your emotional condition now? Are you able to *handle* stress, or is stress *handling* you? Are you at the point of needing a break?
- **Clarify the consequences of stress.** How is stress impacting my life? How is my family responding to my pressure? Is stress affecting my health?
- **Make a plan.** Decide what can change and what cannot. What can change in the way I am living? Do I need to seek help with caregiving? Do I need to spend more time and pay more attention to another area of my life?
- **Put your plan into action.** Convert the idea into tangible steps with set times to measure

progress. If you are not making progress, what needs to change in your plan? Adjust.

- **Accountability.** Accountability can be a powerful tool to augment, putting a plan into action. The accountability partner would be responsible for observing the measurement of progress and the consequences of failing to show progress or rewards when making progress.

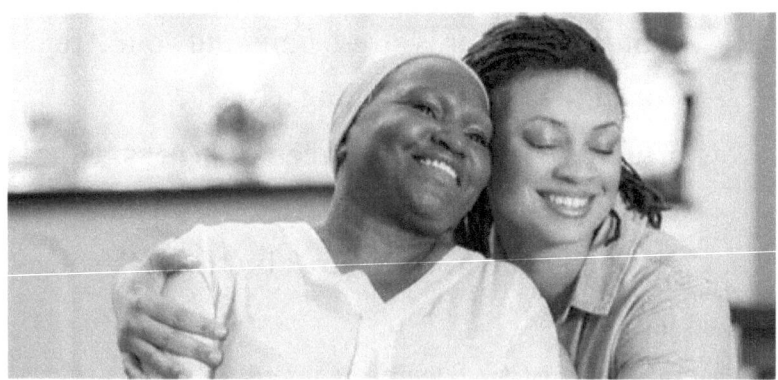

Conclusion

You may be like Martha today and serve as a caregiver. Take these recommendations to heart. Taking on the role of caregiver is indeed noble.

Still, nobility does not make the labor of love immune to exhausting the caregiver and can contribute to several adverse outcomes in the person's life. The overall encouragement is to be in tune with yourself, monitor yourself, and not be dishonest with yourself.

Recognize that caregiving is ultimately a family endeavor. The entire family is responsible for providing the necessary resources to care for the client, including the caregiver.

The place to begin is with a self-care plan. As you review the limitations and weaknesses confronting you, what activities could be helpful?

- Practice calming and stress-reduction techniques (deep breathing, yoga)
- Do not ignore healthcare needs
- Get proper rest and nutrition.
- Create an exercise routine that you will follow.

- Take time off without feeling guilty.
- Find and participate in activities that you enjoy and re-energize you, like going for walks or reading.
- Request and accept support from others.
- Acknowledge your feelings and explore your thoughts that led to these feelings.
- Look for the positives

Lastly, you can do this. Take care of yourself. Perhaps the Golden Rule might be helpful. Treat them the way that you want to be treated.

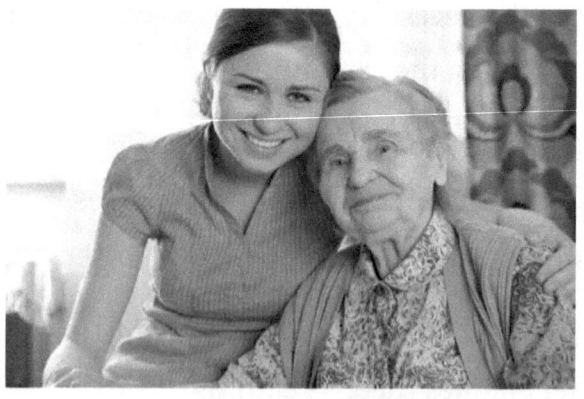

Author Note

Dr. Grice is a licensed professional counselor, educator, and ordained minister. Dr. Grice is a published author and works with families touched by trauma and traumatic loss.

Final Thoughts

I hope the book was a benefit for you. If you have questions, feel free to contact me at mccsdothan@gmail.com

Please leave a review of the book.

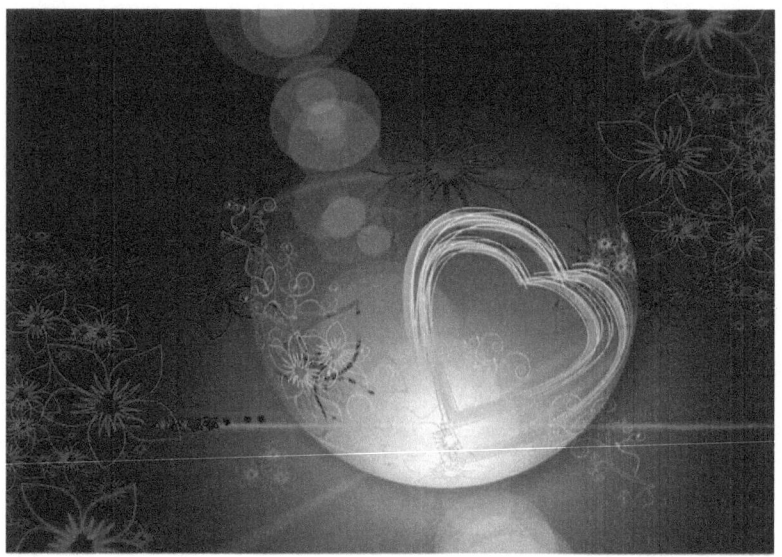

www.ingramcontent.com/pod-product-compliance
Lightning Source LLC
Chambersburg PA
CBHW030545220526
45463CB00007B/2983